Beauty Bath

How to Create a Professional Quality Home Spa for Relaxation and Pure Indulgence

Ruth Logan

ISBN-13: 978-1517765651
ISBN-10: 151776565X

CONTENTS

BEAUTY BATH

INTRODUCTION

Glare at the clock.

Dash into the bathroom and turn on the taps to fill the bathtub and dash out.

Glare at the clock.

Tear all the clothes off your body.

Dash back in to check the temperature and glare at the clock again before shutting the bathroom door.

Grab a random handful of bath supplies and get into a half-filled tub that has water that is either too hot or too cold.

Finish up in the shortest possible time and dash out and glare at the clock.

Does this scenario sound painfully familiar? If it does, it's probably because it is exactly what we all do on a regular basis. Even on the days when we are determined to not just 'grab a quick shower' and decide to relax in a hot bath, the reality usually follows the pattern described above. As a result, we are no less stressed than we were before the 'relaxation effort' and have also harmed our skin in the process, by subjecting it to harmful water temperatures and harsh treatment.

So why does it happen? One clear reason is the sheer lack of precious minutes that are required to take a rejuvenating and refreshing bath. This is why the clock becomes the most important aspect of this activity. The second and more serious reason is a lack of knowledge about the amazing benefits of a proper bath. Most people ignorantly assume that the only purpose of a bath (like that of a shower) is to just get clean in the shortest time possible. It is the desire to dispel this ignorance that is at the heart of this book. There is a truly mind boggling array of benefits to taking a thorough and relaxed bath. What's more, the benefits are certainly more than skin deep! A perfect Beauty Bath can significantly alter a person's mood, relaxation and sense of well-being for the better. Physically and emotionally, something as simple as an indulgent soak can prove to be a powerful antidote to fatigue, pain, stress and general irritability.

As you pore over the pages of this book I hope that you will allow the contents to permeate deep within you. I hope that you will allow these ideas and thoughts to infuse a sense of joy and health into your bath time rituals and that you will protect that time as something precious and essential to your happiness and quality of life.

CHAPTER 1 – THE MANY BENEFITS OF BATHING

A common misconception is that taking a bath is like driving in and out of a car wash. At a very basic level, this is definitely factual. However, with a little bit of planning, getting clean can be one of the add-on benefits of bathing. There is an astonishing array of benefits both physical and psychological, to taking a leisurely and relaxed bath. How many of these do you know already?

Healing from pain

Soaking in a hot bath induces relaxation at a deep-muscle level. The benefit of this is almost equal to that of a massage and works wonders to alleviate tension headaches and muscular cramps. Relaxed muscles are more elastic and in order to enhance the benefit, just practice some gentle stretches when your body is still warm from the bath. This will gradually correct alignment and position problems and can even eliminate the need for long-term treatments such as offered by a chiropractor!

Healing from disorders

Bathing aids in the healing process by increasing the rate of blood circulation. When damaged tissues have a better supply of blood, they have an improved supply of nutrients which speeds up recovery. This allows the normally humble habit of getting into a bathtub to play a role in the healing of serious disorders such as eczema. In order to maximize the effects of bathing to combat eczema, add about a pound of baking soda to a warm tub of water. Sit back and soak it in for 15-20 minutes. The baking soda will act as an antiseptic and help to open up pores and soothe the skin.

Skin Health

Yeast infections will benefit from cider vinegar added to a warm bath. Vinegar restores the acidic and alkaline balance within the body by just relaxing in the tub! Bathing is also an inexpensive and comfortable way to keep the skin looking young and supple. The soaking makes it easier to slough off dead skin cells and keep the body clean and healthy. Bathing also boosts the skin softening powers of oatmeal, to calm inflamed and itchy skin. Just fill a clean sock with whole oats and seal the open end with a knot or rubber band. Put the sock into the warm water and get a good soak for about 15 – 20 minutes. Your skin will thank you for it.

Overcome Insomnia

Bathing is a well-known cure for insomnia. Soaking in warm water increases the body temperature. When you get out of the bath, your skin cools and this causes the brain to release the melatonin hormone which regulates the body's sleep and waking cycles. As a result, within a short while after a bath, you will find that you are ready to go to sleep.

Healthy Body

A scientific study published in the New England Journal of Medicine points to the benefits of bathing, for people suffering from diabetes. A diabetic who sits in a tub of hot water for just 30 minutes can reduce blood sugar levels by as much as 13%. This takes place when blood vessels become dilated and expand because of the hot water and this improves blood circulation, which in turn allows the body to use insulin more effectively. Another study conducted in Japan established that sitting for as little as ten minutes in warm water caused cardiovascular function to improve in both men and women and enabled them to perform better on exercises. Author Suzi Grant, member of the British Association of Nutritional Therapists states, "I heartily recommend bathing. It can prevent colds and viruses, reduce stress, improve sleep, strengthen blood circulation, boost the immune system and detoxify the body."

A full bath, despite all its many benefits, may not be something you can enjoy on a regular basis. So it is comforting to know that many of the benefits mentioned above can be gained with just a foot bath. A foot bath just requires the feet and legs to mid-calf height to be immersed in water. Add peppermint, lemon or thyme oil to a warm foot bath, soak for about 20 minutes and you will see headaches, colds and achy feet disappear without a trace. Foot baths also help with insomnia. Soak your feet in water as cold as you can bear it for as long as you can bear it. A few minutes later you are sure to be pleasantly surprised by your drooping eyelids. Alternating between hot and cold foot baths is among the most effective techniques to boost blood circulation and help with varicose veins. Soak your tired and unhappy feet in hot water for about two minutes. Then immediately dip them in cold water for about 30 seconds. Keep at this technique for about 15 minutes and make sure you end with the cold water. Sit back and enjoy your feet that are pink and tingling with refreshment.

Psychological

Adding essential oils to bath water can cause significant changes to your moods and feelings. Lavender or eucalyptus essential oils have tried and tested capabilities to reduce stress. A long and peaceful bath with one of these added is sure to ensure a tranquil mental state and a good night's sleep. Sage oil is said to be a great memory and mood booster. Other essential oils such as lemon and orange can awaken the senses and get you revved up for a day of activity. A few drops of oils such as rose and sandalwood in the bath, lightly perfumed, is great for the skin and makes it beautifully soft.

The scientific journal 'Complementary Therapies in Medicine' has stated that taking a warm water bath every day for eight weeks consecutively is better at reducing anxiety levels than taking a prescription drug.

CHAPTER 2 – A QUESTION OF TEMPERATURE

Finding the correct temperature for a bath can sometimes be a matter of life and death. The Royal Society for the Prevention of Accidents estimates that every year, 600 people suffer serious injuries as a result of bathwater accidents because of extremely high temperatures with about twenty fatalities. This unusually high number is mostly restricted to people from demographic groups who cannot bathe themselves such as small children and the elderly who are under the care of secondary or tertiary caregivers. Consequently, it is always important to check and regulate the temperature of a bath before the water comes in contact with your skin. While hot water has its benefits, scalding or freezing water can be counterproductive to a healthy bathing experience.

Accidents involving scalding bathwater often cause lasting damage to the skin and may require surgery to repair the damaged skin and muscle tissue. Burn victims often endure years of painful healing and skin grafts before being able to return to any resemblance of normality. It is said that the late Princess Margaret suffered burns caused by scalding bathwater while holidaying on the island getaway of Mystique in the West Indies, requiring half a year to recover from her ordeal. Hot water from residential taps or solar-powered heaters can go up to 158 degrees Fahrenheit (F) and can cause second-degree and third-degree burns that can be fatal to infants and some children. Even with a temperature regulator, tap water is usually at nearly 122 degrees Fahrenheit, hot enough to cause damage to the skin and remove a layer of the epidermis and sebaceous oils that protect you from bacterial infections and many serious and painful conditions associated with dry skin.

So how do you check the temperature of bath water? A simple rule of thumb is that if the water is too hot for your hand, then it is probably too hot for your body. The skin on your palms is thicker than several other parts of the body, but is equipped with temperature sensors that can easily identify if a liquid is too hot or too cold in a matter of seconds. An even better thermometer than the hand is the inside of the wrist or the elbow. However, be very careful before testing bath water with these parts of the body as the skin there is very delicate and can easily burn. A study by a multidisciplinary research group in Japan has identified that the body undergoes a phenomenon known as heat stress when exposed to high temperatures in the bathroom. So, it benefits you to keep your bathwater at an optimum temperature, but what is this temperature

Optimum Bath Temperature

One of the theories about the optimum temperature of a bath concludes that bathwater needs to be as close to the natural temperature of the human body as is possible, or about 98 degrees Fahrenheit. The theory advances that such a temperature mimics the warmth of the womb and is believed to be particularly comforting for children. However, the water in a shower or in a tub loses temperature as a result of simple heat transfer and rapidly drops in temperature. So, keeping your bath at half a degree or a maximum of two degrees above 98 degrees Fahrenheit can give you all the benefits of a hot bath with none of the harmful effects to worry about.

Above a temperature of 102 degrees Fahrenheit, the body responds to the high temperatures by sending blood to the surface of the skin and away from the internal organs, placing stress on your heart by raising its pulse rate. The effect of this phenomenon is far more pronounced in the elderly and in patients who suffer from compromised cardiovascular or pulmonary function. The Hydrotherapy Association of Chartered Physiotherapists has established that bathwater that is even two and a quarter degrees warmer than your core body temperature can increase your heart rate by 12 percent.

Keeping your bathwater hot can be stimulating and can induce healthy sweating but prolonged exposure to high temperatures in the bathroom can leave you exhausted as a result of life-giving blood being drawn away from joints and muscles. Similarly, sustained exposure for a long period of time to extremely cold water can cause hypothermia and exhaustion as your body shivers to try and maintain its core temperature. However, a quick blast of cold water as part of your shower can invigorate you, closing your pores and preventing you from sweating just as you step out of a bath. Cold water does wonders for the hair, giving it a wavy shine that comes as a result of the closure of the cuticles, according to stylist Daniel Hersheson. Athletes also use cold water to give their muscles a burst of energy and prepare them for a practice session or an event.

Types of Baths

There are several types of baths that offer a variety of benefits just based on the temperature of the water used.

Warm Detox Baths

Keep your bathwater in the range of 90 to 97 degrees Fahrenheit for a luxurious soak that lasts about 15 minutes. This warm bath can improve circulation, lower elevated blood sugar levels, induce a healthy sweat, and relax the muscles. The warmth of such a bath is calming and leaves you with a sense of wellbeing.

Cold Stress Baths

To be avoided by patients with a heart condition, this bath at 54 to 64 degrees Fahrenheit does just the opposite of a warm bath. It invigorates you by helping to increase your blood sugar and shocking the muscles into action. This bath should only last for a few seconds at best, not exceeding half a minute in duration, to avoid the onset of hypothermia and shivering.

Alternate Temperature Baths

Alternating between warm to hot water and cold water is a recent development in hydrotherapy that gives you the best of both types of baths. Favored by athletes for accelerating the healing process, alternating temperature baths can help improve circulation and reduce swelling after intense physical activity.

And so, we see that choosing the temperature of your bath needs to be in consideration of several factors such as your general health, any pre-existing skin sensitivities and a clear understanding of the physical and psychological effects of various bathwater temperatures. For the daily bath, keeping your bath temperature at around 98 degrees Fahrenheit and ending the occasional bath with cold water can do wonders for your wellbeing and appearance!

CHAPTER 3 – THE SPA AT HOME

Creating the perfect environment is essential in order to get a great sense of relaxation and rejuvenation out of a bath. Factors such as harsh or inadequate lighting, frequent interruptions and not having the correct supplies can make taking a bath fraught with aggravation and stress. A lot of work and planning can be undone by the smallest eventuality or a sudden interruption. Follow these simple steps and enjoy an out of this world bathing experience.

Create the space

Tell your family that you do not wish to be disturbed and lock the bathroom door if you have to. Make sure there are no telephones around and close the windows if you have noisy neighbors. Do a quick clean-up of the countertops and mirrors so that your bathroom is transformed into a beautiful place. Adjust the temperature and lighting in the bathroom so that it is exactly the way you like it best. Take your time with the light settings as too much or too little light can ruin a bath. If there isn't much flexibility, use just one or two strategically placed lamps or tall candles. Bring in a music player and put on a playlist of songs that will not require you to get out of the tub to change CDs. Scatter smaller candles or tea lights around the room in safe locations and near the edge of the tub

Add some special touches

Get ready to transport yourself to a place of luxury and indulgence. Keep favorite or luxury foods such as chocolate covered strawberries, gourmet chocolates, a glass of wine, your favorite book or magazine or whatever else your taste runs to, within easy reach while you are in the tub. Roll out a fluffy bath mat so that you don't have to step out onto a cold and slippery bathroom floor. If you have to, buy a new bath towel that is huge, in your favorite color and the best brand that you can afford. Also invest in a silk or fluffy cotton robe so that you continue to feel pampered even after the bath and allow the sense of comfort to linger as long as possible.

Gather all your supplies

Make sure that once you are in your bath tub you have no reason to leave it, till you are done. This means having all your bathing supplies stored around you in baskets that can be reached from the comfort of your bubbly cocoon. Dig out that expensive or designer bottle of bathing crème or gel that you have been hoarding. It is all the better if it is part of a set that includes bath salts, a bubble bath, shampoo and moisturizer. The olfactory sense or sense of smell plays a big role in triggering happiness and relaxation. So having a range of bath products in your favorite scent or in scents that aid relaxation such as jasmine and lavender can boost the effectiveness of your at home spa bath. If you intend to keep your hair dry, make sure that you have pins, bands and a shower cap where you can reach them easily. Keep a bottle of chilled drinking water and a cool face towel within easy reach as the hot and steamy air in the bathroom can get you dehydrated and thirsty after a short while. Remember to drink water at frequent intervals so that you do not feel ill or get a headache.

Prepare yourself

If you do not want to spend time actually washing your body in the bath, you can take a quick shower before your bath. If you have the time, you can also go through all your normal routines such as shaving or waxing your arms and legs, shaping your eyebrows etc. These simple steps and the investment of a few extra minutes will ensure that when you walk out of your bathroom, you are equally prepared for a night on the town or to just curl up and go to sleep.

Prepare your bath

If there is one thing that all the experts agree on, it is that the most relaxing and comfortable bath temperature is about two degrees higher than the normal body temperature. So a temperature range of 98 to 102 degrees Fahrenheit should be about perfect. Test the temperature with your wrist and not the hand, as the wrist is a better indicator of how the water will feel when you are in it. Make sure that you stir the water with your hand so that there are no cold or hot pockets and the temperature is uniform. Whether you are using a bubble bath or a scented bath oil, start pouring it in just under the water flowing from the tap and when the tub is about half full. This will help to disperse the product well into the water with minimal effort from you and in no time you will have an inviting tub to slip into. Scented oils or essential oils are great mood altering agents. If your bath is the first step to enjoying a night out, use scents that will stimulate and sharpen your senses. Alternatively, if it is the first step to a cozy and quiet evening at home or in bed, pick floral scents that will help you unwind and relax.

Luxuriate in an exquisite experience

Place an anti-slip mat at the bottom of the tub to give you greater control of how you want to sit or lie down. Place a small cushion or even better, a warmed and rolled up cotton towel under your neck to support your neck and head comfortably on the edge of the tub. Just sit back and inhale the steam, the scents and the listen to the sounds around you. Let the water and heat penetrate deep into your skin and work their magic. Don't feel like you have to be doing something every minute you are in the tub. Take your time and restrict your movements to the minimum in the first few minutes. Consciously slow down every action and slow your breathing rate so that your mind gets the signal that it is safe and fine to relax.

A little bit of preparation and effort will work wonders to give you an amazing experience that you will soon become addicted to. As you do it more often, you can get more creative and add your unique touches to personalize your perfect bath.

CHAPTER 4 – TO SCRUB OR NOT TO SCRUB

So you are in the tub, all relaxed and happy, the music is playing, the water feels just right, now what? The easiest way to glowing and radiant skin after a hot bath is to use a sponge or loofah to gently exfoliate and remove all the dead skin cells from the skin surface. This brings us to the question of which products to buy. Are you puzzled about finding the best products out of the bewildering choice of soaps, washes, gels, loofahs, sponges and brushes that are available? Read on to get valuable tips and guidance.

The best way to remove dead skin cells is to gently scrub them away. This is easy with the help of specialized bathing tools such as loofahs, sea sponges and various kinds of brushes, pumice stones and scrubbers. Back scrubbers with all-natural bristles are especially effective at clean the back all the way down. You can also use them for other hard to reach areas such as the soles of your feet, toes and ankles.

Loofahs

The most easily available is the common loofah and it's the variety that is the best choice for regular or even daily use. It retains its shape even when soaked in water and is very easy to clean and quick to dry. The Egyptian loofah, which is sometimes called the Luffa is the largest variety. In its native form, it can sometimes be as big as 25 inches long. It is more loosely knotted and less dense than the common variety, which makes it much easier to handle in the bath. The Mayan loofah offers the best middle ground in terms of density and softness and is usually available in 10 inch sizes. Back scrubbers, facial pads and facial discs can also have loofah surfaces, but these must be used with caution to avoid damaging the delicate facial skin.

Sea Sponges

This is another useful bathing tool which can remove dirt and dead skin without damaging the pores. Sea sponges sometimes have other materials added to them as part of the manufacturing process. This allows them to be available in a range of colors and sizes. The texture can range from the entirely natural, to sponges that are as soft as silk or somewhere in between. The size that is the most easy to use is about 5 or 6 inches but larger ones of 7 inches and more also work well for a luxurious effect. If you can find a large uncut sea sponge, it will make for a very unique and special bathing experience. Use it as the basis for a bath with an ocean theme, with some seashells for décor and a soundtrack of ocean waves and falling water.

According to Dr. Jami Miller, MD, an assistant professor in the dermatology department of the Vanderbilt University Medical Center in Nashville, Tennessee, buying bath products is for the most part, guided by personal preference. She cautions against falling for the traps set by celebrities and advertisements and urges people to base their preference on their skin type – dry, oily, combination, infected, sensitive etc. She also states that certain products work better with warm rather than hot water and that it is very important to moisturize after a bath or shower.

Dr. Miller states that almost all soaps and body cleansers remove natural oils from the skin that keep it moisturized naturally. This leaves the skin dry and flaky. However speaking of the difference between soaps and body washes, Dr. Miller says that body washes and a few soaps that have been specially created for sensitive skin, leave a fine film or layer of oil on the skin which helps to replace the natural oil which has been removed. Non-foaming cleansers also tend to be better at retaining some of the skin's natural moisture, than the body washes that produce a thick and heavy lather.

The world is pretty cleanly divided between bathers who like to be 'squeaky clean' after a bath and those who love their skin to feel soft and silky even after soaking in a hot tub for over an hour. Skin experts such as Dr. Miller caution against the squeaky clean effect for both men and women. Soaps and body washes that provide the feeling of being well scrubbed are much harsher on the skin. They strip away all the natural oils on the skin and offer no replacement. On the other hand, some soaps and body washes leave behind what is commonly called a 'film' on the body. This is a layer of oil that is not easily washed away. This film acts as a moisture barrier and prevents just washed skin from drying out and losing elasticity.

If the idea of emerging from a bath feeling oily is not entirely appealing, try out some of the newest formulations of soaps, and particularly shower gels. Gels tend to not be as heavy as crème washes but still protect the body better than most soaps. This is because they closely resemble skin lipids and therefore are absorbed a lot better by the skin. As far as possible, if your skin does not easily break out, it is good to choose products that will blanket your skin in a layer of protection while you are enjoying your bath. That is the best way to ensure that you get all the enjoyment without any of the worry and damage.

CHAPTER 5 – BODY POSITION

Amazingly, some people find sitting in a tub to be quite uncomfortable. If the tub is at two levels or has an inbuilt seat, this discomfort is not usually a problem. But these kinds of tubs have the disadvantage of not allowing the bather to lie down properly. So how do you get comfortable in a full length, single level tub? Is there a way to get so comfortable that you find yourself falling asleep in about five minutes after getting in? Follow these simple tips and enjoy a safe and injury-free bathing experience!

Good Support

A tub bath can suddenly turn into a dangerous or unpleasant experience, with no warning. This usually happens when your head, a knee or elbow is knocked against the faucets or sides of the tub. Unless you are seated securely and comfortably, there is always the risk of worry, discomfort or even injury. Always ensure that you are seated completely and preferably on an anti-slip mat that has been placed at the bottom of the tub. Ensure that your back is well supported and cushioned with either a thick layer of towels or bath cushions. When you lie back, place a rolled up towel securely under your neck to take the strain off your back and neck muscles. Do not shy away from asking family members for help while getting in and out of the bath.

Eye Care

When your eyes are open they are constantly relaying messages to your brain. This keeps the brain in a constant state of alertness and this is counterproductive to your efforts to get calm and peaceful. The eyes also seldom get the care and pampering that they deserve and are normally worked hard for even 16 hours a day or more. Taking a luxurious bath is an ideal way to get two solutions with one action. First of all, close your eyes. In a matter of seconds, you will find yourself relaxing and your pulse and rate of breathing will slow down to a more normal and healthy rate. If you find it difficult to keep your eyes closed, place thin slices of slightly chilled cucumber over them and layer a wet face towel over that. When you look at yourself in the mirror the next time, you will be pleasantly surprised by those bright and beautiful eyes looking back out at you.

Hands and Legs

As long as you are seated firmly and your head and back are supported, it is perfectly fine to fill enough water to allow your hands and legs to defy gravity for a short while. Enjoy the feeling of floating in the water, as you force your mind let go of all its accumulated stresses and worries. Release the child in you and don't be shy or afraid to splash around in the tub, even if it means that some of the water splashes out. This will also provide some exercise, however minimal. Play any games that you can, make shapes out of the soap suds or pretend you are a celebrity. Just about anything is fine as long as it is not dangerous and you are having fun.

Ensuring that you are well supported and seated correctly can make all the difference between a perfect bath and a complete disaster.

CHAPTER 6 – BEAUTY BATH PRODUCTS

More than anything else in the world, baths are meant to be fun—a time for relaxation and playful enjoyment. Luxuriant baths can be just as therapeutic to the mind as they are for the body and can be used to create a unique personal space that is your own. With a few carefully chosen bath products, a bathroom can become a medieval bathhouse or a cartoon-like play world. Fun bath products can turn the most mundane bath into a wonderful time where the imagination takes flight and fantasies can come to life. Today, a wide range of bath products are designed to make your bathing experience special and importantly, a time for joy and laughter while giving your body the cleansing and the essential nutrients it needs. Let's look at a few bath products.

Bath Salts

Ancient practitioners of medicine have been recommending the use of bath salts for over four and a half thousand years. Bath salts find a reference in some of the early writings of ancient China dating back to 2500 BC and Hippocrates is said to have recommended baths in sea water and scented baths. Today, a variety of bath salts are used along with essential oils and other aromatherapy products. Adding bath salts to a hot tub softens the water and gives it a delicate aroma that lingers on the skin for a long time. Bath salts infused with essential oils can accentuate the aroma of your skin and are used in many cultures to replace artificial alcohol-based deodorants. Bath salts with magnesium compounds are known to have an anti-inflammatory effect, leaving your skin with the gentle radiance of good health. Most bath salts also prevent the skin from absorbing too much moisture. Other bath salts containing magnesium and glycerin have exfoliating and emollient properties, carefully removing dead skin and locking in essential moisture.

When bathing with aromatic bath salts, ensure that the water temperature is only warm, as extremely hot water can adversely alter the properties of these salts. Once you have filled a little water, stir in the salts slowly, without agitating the water and allow the bath salts to gradually dissolve. Once the bath salts dissolve, draw your bath by adding water to balance the aroma and concentration for a luxurious, fragrant bath. You can even make your own bath salts with do-it-yourself kits that contain base salts and essential oils. Bath salts are available in floral, spice, earthy, fruity, and herbal fragrances to suit your mood. Choose a strong floral fragrance such as rose or patchouli for an intense soak or a lighter fragrance such as spearmint or lavender for an ethereal bath experience. Every fragrance and essence has a varied effect on the body. For example, lavender and jasmine are known to have soporific effects, aiding relaxation and sleep while peppermint and lemon are known to have exactly the opposite effect. So choose your fragrance to suit your body's needs.

Body Scrubs

Body scrubs are similar in composition to bath salts, using magnesium salts, phosphates, and common salt but use finer crystals for the purpose of exfoliation. If you are looking to remove that layer of dead skin without ruining your skin's pH balance, a body scrub is an ideal agent. Body scrubs should only be used once or twice a week, as continued exfoliation can cause the epidermis to become sore and open to infection. Body scrubs also contain a higher percentage of moisturizing agents, such as shea butter and cocoa butter and use a variety of natural ingredients such as cocoa, honey, coconut oil, olives, tea, peach, argan oil, jojoba, aloe vera, that impart their natural healing properties and nourishing the skin.

Apply body scrubs liberally and spread them gently. Body scrubs may contain fine crystals of sea salt that are a natural astringent, firming up the skin while natural oils serve to moisturize and protect. Caribbean lime and mint scrubs are known for their rejuvenating properties, leaving your skin feeling fresh while Brazil nut improves circulation just below the surface of the skin. No matter which body scrub you choose, the basic composition consists of a moisturizer, an astringent such as sea salt or common salt, and organic oil such as carrot oil or soy oil that repairs the skin. Body scrubs are usually best used before a bath, working them into the skin to stimulate circulation.

Shower Gels

One of the most common mistakes while using bath salts and pre-bath emollients is to use an ordinary soap to complete your bath. Ordinary bath soaps contain a high concentration of caustic soda and caustic potash. These fairly strong alkalis can reverse nearly all the positive effects of bath salts, robbing the skin of precious nutrients. Antibacterial soaps with triclosan can be even more harmful, drying your skin in minutes. Shower gels are specially formulated to wash away excess oils without stripping away the essential quantity that your skin needs. Feeling squeaky clean may seem healthy for a while, but the depletion of essential skin oils is not beneficial in the long term.

You may notice that most shower gels don't dry your skin out completely but leave you with a slightly oily sensation. This sensation is because of the oil added to the gel to preserve your skin's natural oils. Most shower gels are made of an essential oil, fruit infusions, and a foaming surfactant. The oils of choice include almond, coconut, and olive oils paired with vanilla extract and often reinforced with vitamin E for nourishment. Shower gels can make any bath time fun without damaging sensitive skin. Shower gels shouldn't be left on the skin for more than a few minutes as the detergent properties may begin to dry out the skin. Shower gels are ideal for a quick shower on a busy day while ensuring that your skin does not dry too rapidly.

Bath Bombs

Bath bombs are not just great for your skin; they are loads of fun to watch. A bath bomb is usually shaped like a ball containing citric acid that is found in lemon juice and an effervescent such as baking soda combined with moisturizers and essential oils to produce the perfect fizzy bath. Named after the fizzy effect they produce when dropped into water, bath bombs are a perfect way to have a perfect personalized party in the bath. The natural effervescence of baking soda combines well with the essential oils and added colors can create vibrant patterns on the surface of the water.

Drop a bath bomb gently into the water and allow it to float around for a while. It should begin to fizz in a few seconds and fill your bath with an explosion of color and fragrance. Some bath bombs are infused with the petals of flowers to create a lush floral pattern on the surface of the water while others contain bath salts that invigorate the skin with a continuous effervescence that lasts for the entire duration of your bath. Some of the most popular bath bombs use:

Lemongrass – a subtle oriental fragrance that aids relaxation

Honey – a warm and soothing fragrance that softens the senses

Rose – for a royal bath, strong, potent and intensely feminine

Lavender – One of the herbs that are perfect for a lazy soak before bedtime

Lemon – a fresh, tantalizing fragrance to start the day with

Bath bombs should be handled with care, choosing the products that contain ingredients that match skin and hair type. A bath bomb is a fun treat for children and the elderly, adding a touch of excitement and transforming an otherwise boring chore into a healthy, invigorating experience.

Bath Melts

Often regarded as being complimentary to bath salts, bath melts are a healthy dose of essential and carrier oils best suited to revitalize tired or drying skin. Also known as tub truffles, bath melts are usually made of cocoa butter or shea butter with a single fragrance or a bouquet of essential oils. Parched skin that is in need of repair needs more than the usual volume of oil to return to health and vibrancy. A bath melt works just like a bath bomb, but instead of fizzy and frothy effervescence, it merely melts into a bathtub spreading the goodness of essential oils to create a delightful bathing experience.

Bath melts help to preserve and build up the skin, imparting the essential nutrients it needs to grow and heal. Natural bath melts have several herbal additives and lemon zest extracts with essential oils from fruit or floral extracts. The product is designed to melt when it comes in contact with the body or water that is at 97 degrees Fahrenheit. Bath melts should not be placed in very hot tubs as dissolving the oils too quickly tend to dissipate the aroma. Avoid the use of soap after a bath with a bath melt.

Bubble Bars

Imagine a bubble bath solution that gives you a steady stream of bubbles for the entire duration of your bath. Bubbles bars are designed to release a sustained stream of bubbles that envelop you in a cocoon of bubbly goodness, creating the perfect cloak of lusciousness. These bars are made up of Sodium Lauryl Sulfoacetate (SLSA), essential oils, carrier oils and a perfume. Unlike Sodium Lauryl Sulfate, SLSA does not irritate the skin, cause follicular damage or

Crush your bubble bar and sprinkle it into a tub, agitating the water to create a blanket of bubbles or leave the bar whole so that you can make bubbles whenever you need to. Bubble bars can also be used for multiple baths and like a soap bar, last for weeks when used sparingly but can also be used to create that one exquisite profusion of bubbles that means loads of bath time fun.

Bubble Bath Toys

Children have the unique talent of being able to make toys out of almost anything—including soap. Bubble bath toys combine the properties of a bubble bath, shampoo, and soap with the malleability of playdoh or modeling clay. Keeping a child (or an adult) enthralled during bath time is so much easier with these soft, cleansing products that also contain powerful and dermatologically safe foaming agents. Bubble bath toys don't need to be crushed or sprinkled and can be used exactly as you would use a soap, but produce a bounty of bubbles and contain soothing oils such as almond oil that is rich in vitamin E and the proteins that stimulates the skin while protecting it and giving it a soft, nourished glow. Almond oil is one of the core ingredients in most baby products as the gentle oil protects and moisturizes without blocking your pores.

Bath Foam

When there isn't enough time to spend time lathering and scrubbing, bath foams are the ideal product. Bath foams are formulated in exactly the same ways as shaving foams but contain soothing oils that are safe on hair and skin. Despite a variety of formulations, many bath foams contain calendula, or pot marigold oil that has several anti-inflammatory and other medicinal properties.

Bath foams designed for adults can contain a variety of soothing and revitalizing natural essences such as shikakai, lavender, patchouli, vanilla, gypsophila, and jasmine. When time is a luxury and bath time comes a premium, such as on a busy Monday morning, a bath foam can shave those precious minutes off the clock for you. Most bath foams are also safe for children, leaving them clean from top to toe without having to juggle with soaps, shampoos, and moisturizers.

Investing in the right fun products for your bath can make the experience uplifting. Whether it is the rushed shower before you head off to work, prepare toddlers and children for the day ahead or a luxuriating soak in a warm tub at the end of a tiring day, fun bath products nourish the skin, bringing life and health through a mix of essential oils, skin butters, exfoliating agents and a whole lot of bubbly fun.

CHAPTER 7 – BEAUTY TREATMENTS WHILE BATHING

Sitting in a warm bathtub in a steamy bathroom is a great way to catch forty winks, watch a show, listen to music or catch up on reading. But there are also a whole lot of other activities you can do, to give your entire body, from the top of your head to the tips of your toes, some attention. Hair, facial skin and nails will respond beautifully to specialized treatments because they are already softened by the heat and steam in the room. Here are some things you could try for some extra pampering.

Facials

Who says that spas and salons have the best facials? There are innumerable kinds of facials and specialized treatments you can make and use right from your home. The ingredients for these will cost a fraction of what a commercially produced finished product would. More importantly, you can be sure of the purity and quality of everything in it – something that is never possible in a bought product. Here are a few ideas for luxurious and restorative home facials that you can try.

Never compromise on quality. If you must buy some products for your home facial, buy the best and most natural products. If you have the ingredients at home, never use expired items or anything that seems even slightly off or stale. Ensure that you have whatever you need, neatly lined up within reach of your bath tub. Never bring any electrical appliance such as steamers, facial massage tools etc. near the bath tub.

Ensure that you follow all the steps of a professional facial, to get the best results. Possibly the only step that can be omitted is the steaming because the steam from the bath would have done that for you already. First cleanse your skin and remove all traces of makeup, using a gentle cleanser and cotton balls or a soft cloth. The next step is to exfoliate. Both store bought and homemade scrubs are equally effective at gently removing dead skin and other impurities. Good homemade scrubs can be made by making a paste of cornmeal and organic yoghurt, honey and extra virgin coconut oil, and many other combinations. Follow this up with a mask and when you get out of your bath, remember to moisturize your face too.

Masks

Facial masks work in two main ways to boost skin radiance and youthfulness. They seal in moisture and allow the therapeutic benefits of the ingredients to seep into the skin. Masks provide benefits such as cleaning up impurities, unclogging pores, restoring skin tone, erasing fine lines and dark spots, all of which add up to glowing skin. The simplest kinds of masks only require fleshy fruit such as bananas and papayas to be mashed into a paste and applied to the face. Wash off after about 20 minutes. Other ingredients such as honey, milk and yoghurt can be added to these fruit masks to augment their nutritive value.

Milk by itself is a very nourishing mask. Use full cream milk or make a thick paste using milk powder and a little water. Apply and wash off after it has dried on your face. An oatmeal mask combines half a cup of oatmeal added to half a cup of hot water. After it cools, add 1 tbsp. of honey and 2 tbsp. of plain yoghurt and the white of a small egg. Apply this mixture to your face and rinse off after about 15 minutes, for skin that is pink with health.

Foods such as mayonnaise and yoghurt make excellent face masks by themselves. For an added glow, a little bit of fresh orange juice or the pulp of half an orange can be added to the yoghurt. Mustard is also a good option for a mask, but try a little on a small area of your face first to test for any reaction. Eggs make great masks and are suitable for all skin types. For dry skin, apply just the yolk. If you have oily skin, whip the egg white only and add some lemon and honey. Normal skin will benefit from having the entire egg applied to the face and washed off when dry.

Hair Treatments

Instead of twisting and knotting your hair up and leaving it to sweat under a shower cap while you enjoy your luxury bath, why not give your hair some TLC too. If you have hair that is dry, damaged or prone to dandruff, there is a lot that you can do, while in the bath, that will save time and give you shiny, soft tresses when you step out.

Oils such as castor oil and extra virgin olive and coconut have been the secret of generations of women with long, strong and lustrous hair. Just massage the oil into the hair, leave it on for about 30 minutes and shampoo as usual when you step out of your bath. Foods such as mayonnaise, bananas, eggs, avocado and even beer will also nourish dry hair. Make a paste and apply it from the roots to the tips, wait for 15 20 minutes and wash with a gentle shampoo. Most of these treatments can be done 2-3 times a week.

Oily and lifeless hair too will benefit greatly from some attention in the bath. After shampooing your hair rinse it with a combination of water and apple cider vinegar, tea or lemon juice. Follow this up with a cold water final rinse. Those with blonde hair must avoid using black tea as it can sometimes stain the hair. Green tea is a good substitute. Aloe Vera gel is another good product for oily hair. Mix one cup each of this gel and your shampoo with two tbsp. of lemon juice. You can store this in your fridge for up to a week. Use this twice a week for oil-free bouncy hair.

Hands and Feet

Hands and feet deserve as much pampering as they can get because of all the stress, wear and tear they are put through on a regular basis. While taking a bath is the best time to give yourself a manicure and pedicure so that when you come out, you are ready have some fun painting your finger and toe nails.

First off, clean your nails thoroughly. There is no other way to do this other than to use nail polish remover. Nail polish remover is not good for your fingers, nails or cuticles, even if it claims to contain moisturizers and even if it claims to not contain acetone. The trick is to use as little as possible and never soaking your fingers in it. After removing the polish, cut the nails and file them into the shape you like. A crystal file is the gentlest on the skin because it will not tear the nails or harm the cuticles. Avoid metal emery boards or ones that are too rough. Keep your nail shape somewhere between practical and beautiful and resist the urge to shape them into long talons. Toenails must be cut carefully and in a straight line just a little bit away from the skin. If you cut them too short, you will have a good chance of developing ingrown toenails. Soak your hands and feet in little bowls of water or simple let them soak in the tub, after you have cut and shaped your nails and not before. Soaking them before cutting makes them weak and susceptible to damage while filing.

Cuticles can be moisturized with a very thick moisturizer. These work just as well as any cuticle cream and the latter do not do anything very beneficial for your nails or cuticles. A good polish or scrub will take years of your fingers and toes. A simple scrub can be made with some organic oil and a little sugar. Avoid the temptation to brutally scour the skin as these will stretch and damage the skin. Use gentle circular movements to work the scrub into the skin and then rinse off with warm and then cold water. A foot file or pumice stone will make it easy to remove the tougher skin and calluses from your feet.

To make your finger and toe nails appear longer and well defined, push the cuticles back from the nail, all around the edges. This must be done very slowly and gently so that the cuticle does not tear and normal nail growth is not affected. Do not use any force or attempt to lift the cuticle in any way. Gently trim any stray bits of cuticle that are sticking out but do not cut near the nail bed. Ideally do the manicure and pedicure in the last few minutes of your perfect bath. This way, as soon as you are done, you can get out of the bath and slather on the moisturizer.

Massages

Another luxury activity that will save you a lot of money and can be done during a bath is to give yourself a good massage. Here are some simple guidelines.

Head

A scalp massage will immediately relax you and drain away the tensions and anxiety in your mind. Just place the heels of your palms on your temples and gently push the skin toward the ceiling, hold for 10 seconds and release. Work your way over your entire head in a similar manner.

Face

Begin at your hair line and draw light circles all along it, coming down to the cheekbones, eyebrows and the edge of your jaw. Avoid working around the edges of your mouth and near the eye area as the skin is thin and delicate. Massage your ear lobes and ears with the tips of your fingers.

Hands and arms

Give your hands a gentle massage by placing one arm on your thigh with the palm facing upward. Use the heel of your other hand to gently push down on your arm, in the direction of your wrist. Continue with this movement all across the palm and to the tips of each finger. Repeat this action over the mound of your thumb and again about three times for the same arm before switching to the other arm.

Neck and shoulders

A long warm bath will have considerably loosened the muscles of your neck and shoulders, providing relief from pain and tightness. To make that benefit go even further, give your neck a good stretch by slowly lowering your chin to your chest. Place your fingertips at the point where your neck and shoulders meet and press firmly. Hold till you feel your shoulders relaxing and then release. Then slowly roll each shoulder back and forth. Repeat all these steps till you feel perfectly loosened up and relaxed.

Lower Back

Wedge a smooth massage roller or even just a clean tennis ball between your back and the bath tub. Slowly slide your body in up and down and side to side movements and let the warm water and the ball loosen up those muscles that are tight with fatigue and stress. Press hard enough to feel pressure but not so much so as to cause any pain and do this only for about two or three minutes in order to not damage the skin.

Thighs, calves and feet

Use the same tennis ball and or massage foam roller to just roll away the pain and tension from your thighs. Alternatively you can just use your elbow by leaning forward and running your elbow in light and firm strokes all the way along the thigh, right down to your knees. Use different angles to cover as much of the thigh as possible. Calves tend to tighten up for various reasons such as standing for too long or wearing high heels for extended periods. Relax your tired calf muscles by pressing or dragging the heels of your hands from your foot to your knees. Flex your foot as you do this and feel the sense of well-being that will envelop you. Give your toes a work out by gently bending them forward and backward and rotating them both clockwise and counterclockwise.

CHAPTER 8 – BATHING AND YOUR MIND

A bath is not just a mundane activity that needs to be accommodated in your day. Since ancient times, bathing has been an activity that is both a sign of good health and an activity designed to benefit the mind as much as it brings relaxation to the body. More often than not, bathing is relegated to being a cursory chore, with no mental preparation or consideration for the effect that a bath can have on your mind. However, this phenomenon is a modern one as most ancient cultures instituted elaborate rituals surrounding a bath that prepared the body and the mind. Even today, bathing is a therapeutic form of physical cleansing; one that finds resonance with several disciplines of mental health associated with meditation and relaxation techniques. The catchphrase, "A nice warm bath and a good book" as a means to calm the nerves has become something of an urban cliché that now has scientific backing.

A study by researchers at Yale University has established a relationship between bathing, mental health and social connectedness, postulating that a warm, relaxing bath has positive effects on the mind, helping people stave off loneliness.

Preparation

In ancient Japan, a bath was preceded by much preparation. Bathing implements were carefully placed, a session of meditation and massage preceded the bathing ritual, and every traditional bath was designed to be a cornucopia of sensory pleasure, ensuring that every one of the senses was presented with stimuli that would relax the body and the mind. Running out of soap or an inaccessible towel was unheard of in ancient times, as laying out bath implements and after-bath treatments was one of the key aspects of preparation. The modern bather has many accessories that can prepare the mind and body for a refreshing and revitalizing experience, and can learn a great deal from the bathing practices of the past.

Meditation

Bath meditation is one of the most powerful techniques to deal with stress triggers and greatly magnify the benefits of a relaxing bath. You may choose to use any meditation technique before your bath and during a long soak in the tub. Meditating in the lotus position under a shower is one of the best-kept secrets of modern practitioners of meditation technique that mirrors the oriental technique of meditating beside or under a gentle stream of falling water. Meditation techniques and visualization have been proven to be powerful tools that boost cognitive and emotive function, and a bath is the perfect setting to

Aromatherapy

Hydrotherapy and aromatherapy have a storied association that dates back to the ancient Egyptian, Greek, Chinese, Japanese, Indian and Persian civilizations. Water used for bathing was often infused with herbal, floral and fruit essences in addition to salts and minerals to combine the potent benefits of both disciplines. In the modern setting, bath melts and aromatherapy candles can help relieve stress, induce the relaxation of tired muscles, and even act as an aphrodisiac. The aroma you choose for your bath can be used to set the mood and influence your mind. A study published in Chemical Senses indicates that fragrances have a powerful influence on the mood and physical wellbeing irrespective of age.

Relaxation – Soothing herbs such as patchouli, sandalwood, ylang ylang, rose and jasmine create an environment that enables your mind to settle into a restful state, dissipating stress by the sustained release of endorphins, the hormones responsible for relaxation. Lavender has been known to induce sleep and is used on conjunction with other relaxing aromas.

Invigoration – Eucalyptus, tangerine, lemongrass, cedar, bergamot, citronella and peppermint are some of the fragrances that are uplifting and refreshing. Consequently, these are ideal for when you want to elevate your mood. Rosemary and Juniper are also stimulating fragrances that combine well with an energizing bath experience without causing undue stress.

Snacking

Medical professionals usually do not recommend eating a heavy meal during a bath. However, a light snack during a bath isn't unheard of and can do wonders for your mind. Tangerines, cheese, carrot sticks, chocolate, crackers and other small snacks that aren't messy can tantalize your taste buds and can be used to complete your bath time experience. Some dieters recommend bath time snacking as a way to reduce portions and control the urge to binge.

Music

Auditory stimulation is one of the commonly overlooked aspects of a bath and the music you choose to listen to can have a significant effect on your mood. The U.S. National Library of Medicine has established the positive effects of soothing music on elderly patients suffering from dementia. Calming sounds such as the sound of running water, rain or the gentle sounds of the wind blowing set to strings, flutes and other warm, rounded and mellow sounds can form the perfect accompaniment to a long soak before bedtime. Ambient, neo-classical, synth-pop and progressive electronic music are believed to be the appropriate accompaniment to a morning shower when you need your senses to be at their peak.

Combining sensory elements with meditation is a powerful way to attune your mind and body while enhancing the intensity of your bath experience. Creating a stress-free environment and using the appropriate combination of fragrance, oils, food, and music can transform a bath into an exquisite confluence where mind and body are healed.

CHAPTER 9 – AFTER-BATH CARE

Finally it's time to end those hours of bliss and luxury and get out of the bath tub. Try not to rush headlong into any heavy and frenzied activity. Take time to correctly dry off and give yourself all the time you need in order to extend and get the maximum benefit out of your perfect bath.

Body

Step into the shower for a quick rinse down first with cool water and then with cold. This will remove all traces of your bath products and also close the pores. Use a soft cotton towel with a high thread count to dry your body. Try to completely dry yourself before stepping out of the room. The humidity will ensure that you don't have to scrub yourself dry and your body will have time to cool and come back to its normal temperature. Use long gentle strokes while drying off and pay special attention to areas with delicate skin, skin folds, in between the toes etc. After the initial wetness has been reduced, try and complete the drying using a blotting action instead of a brisk rubbing down.

Ideally, while still in the bathroom, slather on generous amounts of your favorite moisturizer everywhere on yourself except your face and head. Really work the cream or lotion into your skin with firm and smooth strokes. Pay special attention to the normally dry areas such as your elbows, knees, neck, hand and feet and when you are done, slip into a soft robe. If your face is fresh from an in-bath facial, apply generous quantities of your face cream and massage till it is fully absorbed. If not, clean your face with some astringent to close the pores and then moisturize.

Hair

When you are taking care of your body, if you have washed and conditioned your hair, wrap your wet hair in a dry and warm cotton towel. Try not to wrap it too tightly and have just enough tightness to hold it in place. Find a sunny corner and undo your towel. Dry your hair with a blotting action. Try not to vigorously rub your hair as this can cause the follicles to break or the scalp to become too dry and begin to itch or produce dandruff. When your head is about 70 percent dry, towel the length of your hair. When the hair is more damp than dry, it can be left to air dry the rest of the way.

Gently run your fingers through your hair to detangle it. Never brush or comb wet hair as this will cause the shafts to break. Try not to tie it up or strain your hair in any way. Preferably leave it loose and do a cool-air blow dry if you want to set it. Apply some warmed fragrant hair oil or anti-frizz serum to the tips for added shine and perfectly untangled and silky soft hair in the morning. If you did not wash your hair during the bath, just gently run a wide toothed comb through it and leave it loose and unhindered as you enjoy the rest of your evening.

Nails and Toes

Your beautifully manicured nails and pedicured toes are sure to be crying out for some attention now. Invest in a good quality hand and foot cream to keep dry and cracked extremities at bay. Give your hands and feet a good massage with the cream. Use gentle and firm movements and cover every part. Enclose the fingers in the palm of the other hand and rub the cream in using a gently twisting motion. This will also improve circulation. Link the fingers of both hands together to apply the cream to the spaces in between the fingers. Massage each toe separately and pay special attention to your ankles and heels.

After the cream has been entirely absorbed into the skin, it is time to start coloring! Pick out your favorite shade of nail polish and settle into your favorite chair. Apply a thin base coat and let it dry completely. To get the most professional look, paint one smooth strip down the middle of the nail and then one each on either side. After the base coat has dried, apply two more coats in the same way, waiting for each to dry before starting the next. Finally apply a top coat to get the maximum depth and shine. Let each layer dry naturally. Using a dryer or any other product will not only damage your nails, it can sometimes cause the polish to lift and expand, making it look quite unsightly.

Food and drink

An average person burns between 40 and 85 calories for every hour spent bathing. Soaking in a hot tub for over 20 minutes also causes you to lose water, leaving you hungry for a quick snack. A hot bath or shower causes a natural drop in blood sugar that can leave you feeling weak or ravenous. When your blood sugar levels drop, your body craves sugar, creating the urge to reach out for a bar of chocolate, ice cream, some carbs or a high-calorie dessert. Resisting the urge to fill up on sugary treats can help you snack healthier after a bath.

After-shower nutrition involves choosing a snack that replaces some of the energy you've lost and giving you a healthy dose of minerals and vitamins. A dry fruit smoothie is a healthy energy snack that combines the natural fruit sugars of raisins and other dried fruit with the goodness of yoghurt. Whipping together a simple fruit smoothie is as easy as adding about 125 g figs, raisins, and dates into about 250 ml of yoghurt and running the mix through a blender till it achieves an even consistency. If you need to satisfy your sweet tooth, adding about 100 ml of sweetened apple juice gives your smoothie a tangy flavor and a lighter consistency. If you prefer a healthier option, create your own spinach smoothie with yoghurt, spinach, some green grapes or mango to taste and enjoy a great vegetable treat Fruit or veggie smoothies make for great after-bath replenishment because they are filling, don't pile on the calories, and are a great way to stay nourished.

Tea and mint sandwiches are another easy snack that's light on the stomach and quick to put together. Keep your tea sugarless and without milk to fully benefit from the antioxidant properties of green tea or the herbal infusions of chamomile tea. Chamomile is known for its medicinal and beauty benefits and is a light, aromatic tea with a fruity flavor. Adding ginger or lemon to your tea can put a spring in your step and even stave off the after-bath sniffles.

Entertainment

Showers at the end of the day can send mixed messages to your body clock. After a warm bath, your body receives all the signals that it should rest, but as the moisture on your skin cools, it gives the body a mild wake-up call, improving your alertness for a brief period. During this period, it is good to wind down again by reading a good book or listening to some soothing music to reorient your body to get ready to sleep.

An afternoon shower can also send you mixed signals. As tired muscles relax, you may want to get a short nap, but playing a video game or listening to some upbeat music can keep your mind alert and ready to tackle the rest of the day. Video games on a smartphone or on a PC are a particularly effective way to keep your mind and reflexes alert and responsive after a bath. If it is at bedtime, soft, soothing music aids in the relaxation process. Recorded white noise or the gentle sounds of rainfall can lull your senses to sleep after a warm bath. Try to avoid books that have complicated or disturbing plots such as thrillers and subjects dealing with the paranormal. Magazines based on food, celebrities, movies, and fashion make for great reading material that will help you wind down and get your eyelids drooping.

Sleep

Sleep is one of the body's most natural responses to a comforting bath. A warm bath a couple of hours before calling it a day can actually make the cooling down process work in your favor, according to researchers at the New York University School of Medicine. Dimming the lights also sends a message to your brain that it is time to sleep. As your environment grows darker, the body secretes Melatonin, a hormone that regulates your sleeping cycle, telling your body that it is time to go to sleep. By contrast, a quick power nap before showering can give your eyes and brain the rest they need after a heavy lunch or in cold and dreary weather. It is important to avoid stimulants such as alcohol, caffeine and nicotine just before you sleep as these chemicals can disrupt your sleep cycle and cause a hangover when you wake up. Installing automated time-based dimmers that activate after a bath, closing the drapes, and using a sleeping mask can avoid light pollution. An after-bath routine can also help your body settle into a pattern it can recognize as the first step to a sound nights' sleep.

SUMMARY

For most of us, the world is spinning too fast. There never seems to be enough hours in the day and everything always has to be done yesterday. Life at every turn is filled with anxiety, worry and sometimes even fear. Deadlines loom, nagging people and sicknesses never go away, and everyone expects the world and gives nothing in return.

In such a scenario, respites are few and far between. Warm, cosy dinners with family and friends, annual holidays etc. are becoming relegated to the realm of memory rather than being a part of life. Time has become the rarest and precious commodity in our lives and the ticking of the clock seems more important than the beating of our hearts.

What is the solution? How can this be fixed? The solutions are simple and just need to be implemented and fiercely protected. Taking care of our own physical and mental well-being and that of others closest to us ranks right at the top of the ways to make our lives better. Simple things like sleeping more and eating healthy, if done consistently, can have a profound effect on our health and happiness.

Personal hygiene and grooming is a big part of being healthy and feeling good about ourselves. Yet is it usually a very neglected aspect of our lives, with scant minutes devoted to activities such as brushing and flossing teeth, grooming our hair or taking a bath. We buy and use products without a second thought about whether they are harmful in the long run, evaluating their ingredients and checking whether there are safer and better alternatives.

This book has given you a detailed narration of the benefits, tips, methods and ideas on how to take the best bath you have ever had. Great care and hours of research have gone into making this a comprehensive and very readable book that is filled with information from end to end. If however, all this remains just a good read and nothing more, the purpose of this book is not met. This book has the potential to be the beginning of a great new style of living and a vastly improved quality of life for you.

Give yourself the special treatment described within these pages. Make this much more than a one-time or annual event. Decide in your mind to set aside time regularly to put the life back into your existence and the spring back into your step and the sparkle back into your eyes. Give your loved ones the best of you, by giving yourself the best that you deserve. In just a few weeks you will see and feel the difference that just a wonderful bath can make in your life. Your skin and air will look and feel better than ever. You will notice that those old aches and pains that have almost become good friends have stopped coming to visit so often. Colds, coughs, inflamed sinuses, headaches and general fatigue and lethargy will begin to be replaced with better sleep and tons of new-found energy. So go on and fill that tub! You will be so glad you did.

ABOUT THE AUTHOR

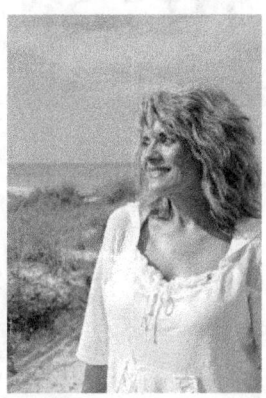

Ruth Logan has been fascinated with Personal Development, Health, and Wellbeing for just over 30 years now. She's particularly passionate about Eastern Philosophy, and the Science behind Wellbeing. Her aim is to share the great benefits of Eastern Philosophy to the unaware in modern society.

Ruth is an avid reader and can't resist learning new information on how we can all better ourselves. Over the last couple of years she's started freelance writing and more recently taken the step to releasing her on work.

In her books, Ruth provides action plans and advice on how to incorporate learning points into 'real life' in a concise yet informative manner.

When not reading or writing, Ruth enjoys walking her dog, cooking and travel.

MORE BOOKS BY RUTH LOGAN

If you enjoyed reading **"Beauty Bath"**, you may like these other books from Ruth Logan.

Gratitude – 7 Simple Steps To Becoming More Grateful In 7 Days

Healing – 7 Ways To Heal Your Body in 7 Days

Learning – 7 Steps To Increasing Your Learning Your Learning Potential In 7 Days

Limiting Beliefs – 7 Ways To Stop Limiting Beliefs In 7 Days

www.ingramcontent.com/pod-product-compliance
Lightning Source LLC
Chambersburg PA
CBHW071134280526
45787CB00003B/1280